Boost Your Metabolism for Sustained Weight Loss

Tips to Speed Up Your Metabolism and Keep the Weight Off

RON KNESS

ISBN-13: 978-1534939752

ISBN-10: 153493975X

Contents

Disclaimer

This publication is for informational purposes only and is not intended as medical advice. Medical advice should always be obtained from a qualified medical professional for any health conditions or symptoms associated with them. Every possible effort has been made in preparing and researching this material. We make no warranties with respect to the accuracy, applicability of its contents or any omissions.

What Is Metabolism?

You've probably heard someone say they can't lose weight because they have a naturally slow metabolism. You may have even said this yourself. Popular diet programs and exercise DVDs promise to *"crank up your metabolism"* for maximum fat burning, weight loss potential. It seems that this thing called metabolism is somehow directly related to losing weight, and healthy weight management.

All of those points beg the question, *"What exactly is metabolism, and is it possible to manipulate it to sustain weight loss?"*

Metabolism is actually made up of 2 different metabolic processes.

> 1) Anabolism - "the set of metabolic pathways that construct larger molecules from smaller units."

> 2) Catabolism – "the process of breaking large molecules down into smaller parts, which are then either oxidized to release energy, or used to create smaller units for the anabolic process."

Anabolic processes can be seen as "building up" tissues, organs and other substances. They create growth in your cells, which in turn increases your body size, musculature, bone structure, etc. You may have heard of anabolic steroids, which promote muscle growth and the synthesis of protein in your body, popular with athletes and bodybuilders.

For example, if you cut your finger, your body (if it's functioning properly) will begin – without even wasting a moment or asking your permission –the process of creating skin cells to clot the blood and start the healing process.

On the other hand, catabolic processes break things down. Proteins, lipids, nucleic acids and other components are deconstructed into amino acids, fatty acids, monosaccharides, nucleotides and other smaller components. Two of the processes of catabolism are to release energy, and to break down larger compounds into simple waste products. Catabolism also breaks down larger substances so that the anabolic processes can reconstruct them into beneficial larger components.

For example, as you aerobically exercise, your body temperature rises as your heart beat increases and remains with a certain range.

As this happens, your body requires more oxygen; and as such, your breathing increases as you intake more O_2. All of this, as you can imagine, requires additional energy.

After all, if your body couldn't adjust to this enhanced requirement for oxygen (both taking it in and getting rid of it in the form of carbon dioxide), you would collapse!

Presuming, of course, that you *aren't* overdoing it, your body will instead begin converting food (e.g. calories) into energy.

Nutrition, Fat, Energy and Metabolism

Your nutrition is the key to your metabolism. The catabolic process has to have something to break down, and it finds these compounds and components in the food that you eat.

This produces energy, which is then used to create new nucleic acids, proteins and other helpful building blocks your body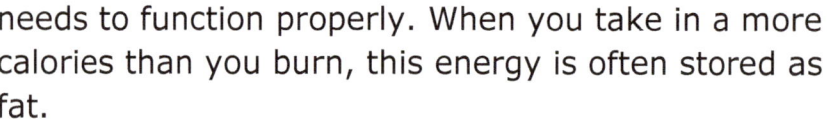
needs to function properly. When you take in a more calories than you burn, this energy is often stored as fat.

When you don't give your body the nutrition it needs, your metabolism is thrown off. You don't create the needed components that lead to proper health.

The metabolic process also works with nutrition to supply the necessary chemicals that your body cannot create on its own.

Fats are nothing more than concentrated sources of energy. Your body needs them, especially since they create 2 times as much energy as either protein or carbohydrates (comparing the same quantity of fat to carbohydrates and protein). Not to mention too that the fat-soluble vitamins of A,E, K and D won't absorb into the body without fat. If your nutrition is poor your metabolic process can lead to unnecessary fat storage and an inability to expose of waste products correctly, which leads to weight gain, overweight and/or obesity in many cases.

Can You Change Your Metabolism?

Doctors used to think your metabolism was dictated by your genetic makeup. If you were born with a slow metabolism, you were more inclined to gain weight. If you have a speedy metabolism, you can eat more, since you naturally burn more calories and fat. While your genes do have something to do with your natural metabolic rate, we now understand that controlling your weight is all about nutrition and exercise.

By eating right and keeping active, you keep your metabolism operating properly. This means unneeded fat and waste products are eliminated instead of being stored as fat, or as poisons and 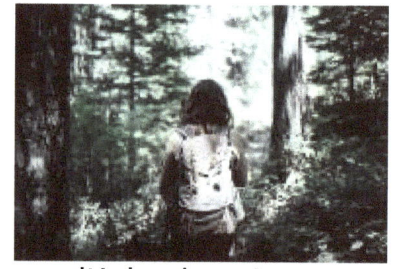 toxins in your liver, leading to multiple chronic conditions. Later in this report you will discover proven ways to boost your metabolism through exercise and nutrition. Now let's take a look at the reason why many diets create a yo-yo weight loss/weight gain situation.

Why Metabolism Slows with Weight Loss or Yo-Yo Dieting

Did you know that losing weight, which seems to be on everyone's mind these days, actually slows down your metabolism? It's true, and it is a natural process that makes sense. If you are skinny and weigh less than average for your height, age and gender, your metabolism should slow down. You don't need as many calories as someone who weighs twice as much as you do, because the energy required to drive all the processes in your body is much less than that other person.

So someone who weighs 150 pounds has a slower metabolism than someone who weighs 200 pounds, on average. This brings us to the problem with fad diets and most other diet plans.

First though, let's take a look at the word diet. Your diet is nothing more than the foods and beverages you eat and drink. Your diet is composed of the nutrients, minerals, proteins, fats, liquids and other components found in the food and beverages you consume. Unfortunately, we have somehow come to understand the word diet to refer to a short-term, low-calorie nutrition plan designed to lose weight.

That is exactly what most diet plans offer – dramatic weight loss as a result of severe calorie restriction. However, that idea is exactly why so many diets show quick weight loss results, followed by even greater weight gain after your diet is over.

Here's what happens.

On a diet, you are told to only eat certain types of foods. You drastically reduce your calorie intake. When you reduce the variety of foods you eat, as well as how much you eat, you usually do not receive the proper nutrition for your body to function properly. Yes, you lose weight, because you are operating at a calorie liability. You are taking on fewer calories than you burn.

However, you are not getting all the nutrients you need to build muscle, and to properly fuel the metabolic process. As your weight goes down, your metabolism naturally drops. At the end of your diet your body is nutritionally starved. So it begs you to eat. You try to return from your diet to a "normal" 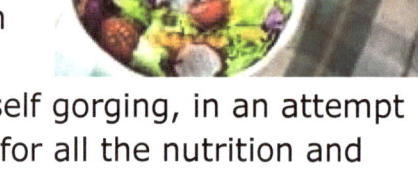 eating plan, but find yourself gorging, in an attempt for your body to make up for all the nutrition and calories it has been missing.

The result? You gain all the weight back that you lost, and in many cases, a lot more.

Just remember, eating too little can slow your metabolism. Your body needs a base number of calories for you to move through your daily routine. When you lose weight rapidly, like on a fad or yo-yo diet, your body thinks it's starving.

It begins burning muscle in place of the calories you are not ingesting, and it also stores fat because it believes you are in starvation mode.

The way to harness your metabolism to lose weight while still being healthy means eating just enough so that you are not hungry, and eating every 3 or 4 hours, several small calorie-count meals throughout the day.

Boosting Your Metabolism with Exercise

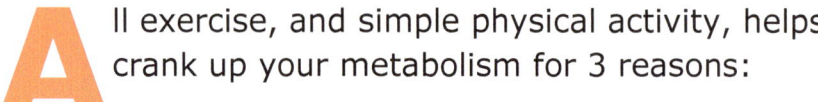

ll exercise, and simple physical activity, helps crank up your metabolism for 3 reasons:

1) exercise builds muscle

2) muscle burns calories at a much faster rate than fat does

3) exercise burns fat instead of muscle for energy, as long as your body is receiving the proper nutrition

When you exercise, when you are physically active, more energy is required than when you are simply sitting. Where does this energy come from? It comes from your metabolic process, which is used to create energy. Exercises that stress your muscles tear them down, and then repairs them bigger and stronger than before. This muscle building process burns a lot of calories, for up to 72 hours after any type of strength training program.

So you can see there is a wonderful cycle of calorie and fat burning which leads to muscle development, which in turn leads to a higher metabolism and even more calories and fat consumed. This is the simple process that physical movement creates.

As WebMD.com puts it so eloquently and succinctly, "Your next workout could set you up for a speedier metabolism."

Since you cannot control your age, your gender and your genetic makeup, common metabolic factors, why not focus on a metabolism influence you do have control over ... **how much exercise you get?** With the aging process comes less muscle mass. This slows down your metabolism, and working out can replace that lost muscle.

Even if you are lazily reclining on the couch watching your favorite reality show, muscle cells burn more energy than fat cells. You have more energy to move through your daily routine when you have more lean muscle mass than fat, you are more mentally sharp and productive, and your metabolism functions at a higher rate. There are so many good reasons for exercising, yet too many people simply don't do enough of it.

What is the best way to use exercise to boost your metabolism? Make your workouts more intense.

You can do this by varying the intensity of your exercise program. This is called interval training. You switch quickly between extremely high and low intensity.

For instance, you may go very hard for 20 or 30 seconds, and then slow down substantially for 10 to 20 seconds. This works great for aerobic exercises like running, jogging or performing Zumba.

You could rip off as many burpees as you can for 1 minute, and then walk for 2 minutes. Repeat this process for 15 or 20 minutes. The idea is to "confuse" your body so that it doesn't know what to expect next. This type of interval training has been shown to burn more calories than static repetitions such as bicep curls or crunches.

Another proven way to fire up your metabolism through exercise is with any type of strength training program.
Remember, muscles burn 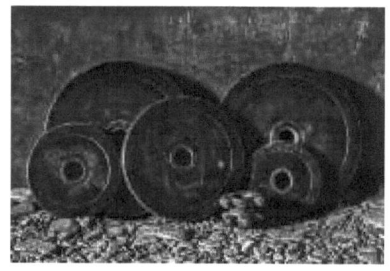 significantly more calories than fat. Also, as you are strength training, you are burning fat and calories, while additionally building muscle. There introduces a wonderful side benefit of strength training ...

Low repetitions with heavy weights deliver the most benefits – this means that significant weight loss and muscle development doesn't take that much time.

Work with whatever weight you can perform for 8 to 12 repetitions, but no more. Then perform 3 sets, 3 to 5 times a week. Make sure to never work the same muscle groups on back-to-back days.

Work your abs, quads, biceps, glutes and other muscles on alternate days. Three sets of 8 to 12 repetitions does not require much of a time investment. However, the muscle rebuilding process, and your metabolism, work for as much as 72 hours after your strength training efforts, which is an incredible weight loss benefit of lifting weights.

What's that you say? You don't own a weight set? No problem, you already have all the weight you need for a muscle building program. Body weight training works to build muscle by using the resistance of your own physical weight against you. Gravity, resistance and your body weight come together in specific exercises to deliver the calorie burning, muscle building benefits of a strength training program, without you having to invest a lot of money on heavy, expensive, bulky free weights.

The takeaway - Make your workouts more intense, integrate interval training into your aerobic exercise plan, and strength train to build muscle. This is the best way to maximize the metabolic process for sustained fat burning and weight loss.

Boosting Your Metabolism Via Diet

A s you saw earlier, nutrition and exercise are 2 metabolic influences you have control over. You just learned how you can add simple exercise programs to your weekly routine to boost your metabolic process.

By now, you already have a sense of how metabolism relates to weight loss (catabolic metabolism, or breaking cells down and transforming them into energy).

To understand this process even more clearly, we can introduce a very important player in the weight loss game: the *calorie*.

Calories

Calories are simply units of measure. They aren't actually *things* in and of themselves; they are labels for other things, just like how an inch really isn't anything, but it measures the distance between two points.

So what do calories measure?

Easy: they measure *energy*.

Yup, the evil calorie – the bane of the dieter's existence – is really just a 3-syllable label for energy.

And it's important to highlight this, because the body itself, despite its vast intelligence (much of which medical science cannot yet understand, only appreciate in awe) does not really do a very intelligent job of distinguishing good energy from bad.

 Actually, to be blunt, the body doesn't *care* about where the energy comes from.

Let's explore this a little more, because it's very important to the overall understanding of how to boost your metabolism, particularly when we look at food choices.

In our choice-laden grocery stores, with dozens of varieties of foods – hundreds, perhaps – there seems to be a fairly clear awareness of what's *good* food, and what's *bad* or *junk* food.

For example, we don't need a book to remind us that, all else being equal, a plum is a *good* food, whereas a tub of thick and creamy double-fudge ice cream is a *bad* food.

Not bad tasting, of course; but, really, you won't find many fit people eating a vat of ice cream a day, for obvious reasons. So what does this have to do with calories and energy?

It's this: while *you and I* can evaluate our food choices and say that something (like a plum) is a healthy source of energy, and something else (like a tub of ice cream) is an unhealthy source of energy, *the body doesn't evaluate*. Really.

It sounds strange and amazing, but the body really doesn't care. To the body, *energy is energy*. It takes whatever it gets, and doesn't really *know* that some foods are healthier than others. It's kind of like a garbage disposal: it takes what you put down it, whether it *should* go down or not.

So let's apply this to the body, and to weight gain. When the body receives a calorie – which, as we know, is merely a label for *energy* – it must do something with that energy.

In other words, putting all other nutrients and minerals aside, if a plum delivers 100 calories to the body, it *has* to accept those 100 calories. The same goes for 500 calories from a (small) tub of ice cream: those 500 calories *have* to be dealt with.

Now, the body does two things to that energy: it either metabolizes it via anabolism, or it metabolizes it via catabolism. That is, it will either convert the energy (calories) into cells/tissue, or it will use that energy (calories) to break down cells.

Now the link between calories/energy, metabolism, and weight loss becomes rather clear and direct.

When there is an excess of energy, and the body can't use this energy to deal with any needs at the time, **it will be forced to create cells with that extra energy.** It has to.

It doesn't necessarily *want* to, but after figuring out that the energy can't be used to do anything (such as help you exercise or digest some food), it *has* to turn it into cells through anabolism.

And those extra cells? Yup, you guessed it: added weight!

In a nutshell (and nuts have lots of calories by the way, so watch out and eat them in small portions…), the whole calorie/metabolism/weight gain thing is really just about excess energy.

When there are too many calories in the body – that is, when there's *too much energy* from food – then the body transforms those calories into *stuff*.

And that *stuff*, most of the time, is fat. Sometimes, of course, those extra calories are transformed into muscle; and this is usually a good thing for those watching their weight or trying to maintain an optimal body fat ratio.

In fact, because muscles require more calories to maintain, people with strong muscle tone *burn more calories* without actually doing anything; their metabolism burns it for them.

This is the primary reason why exercising and building lean muscle is part of an overall program to boost your metabolism; because the more lean muscle you have, the more *places* excess calories can go *before* they're turned into fat.

A Final Word About Fat

There's a nasty rumor floating around out there that fat cells are *permanent*. And the nastiest thing about this rumor is that it's true.

Yes, most experts conceded that fat cells – once created – are there for life. Yet this doesn't spell doom and gloom to those of us who could stand to *drop a few pounds*. Because even though experts believe that fat cells are permanent, they also agree that fat cells can be *shrunk*. So even if the absolute number of fat cells in your body remains the same, their size – and hence their appearance and percentage of your overall weight – can be reduced.

Now let's take a look at smart nutrition moves.

- Start eating more fresh and organic vegetables, fruits, nuts and berries.

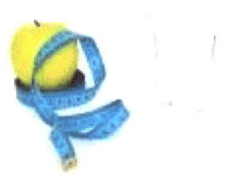

- Drink water throughout the day.

- Eat 5 or 6 smaller meals throughout the day, instead of 2 or 3 large ones.

- Eat some protein at breakfast.

- Eat spicy foods like peppers and Sriracha sauce.

- Choose almond milk over dairy milk.

- Get more whole grains like quinoa, brown rice and oatmeal into your diet, and fewer processed grains like pasta and white bread.

- Eat avocados, peas, pears, figs, artichokes, okra, Brussels sprouts, black beans, turnips and other high fiber foods.

- Eat more egg whites and lean meat.

- Eat celery, a high fiber, low calorie health food that is perfect for filling you up at snack time.

- Fast intermittently. Skip breakfast for 2 days, eating 2 meals around noon or 1 PM, and 7 or 8 PM each day. Then return to 3 regular meals and a couple of healthy snacks on the 3rd day.

- Replace your oils and butter with coconut oil.

- Drink 16 to 24 ounces of water before every meal.

- Drink a cup of coffee, with no cream, milk sugar or artificial sweetener.

- Add cinnamon and garlic to your meals.

- Eat wild caught salmon, a 4 ounce serving 3 or 4 times a week.

- Eat a grapefruit 2 or 3 times a week.

- Drink green tea.

- And seafood to your salad.

- Enjoy all natural Greek yogurt.

- Eat more raw, uncooked foods.

- Eat fewer processed foods (if it comes in a bag, box, can or bottle, it is processed).

Non-Diet, Non-Exercise Ways to Boost Your Metabolism

Is it possible to increase your metabolic rate in some way other than diet or exercise? Working out and eating right are always going to be the smartest and healthiest ways to boost your metabolism and maintain a healthy body weight. However, there are some other things you can do to crank up your calorie and fat burning process.

- Work at a standing desk. Sitting for more than 6 hours a day takes years off your life and substantially increases your risk of dying from any factor.

- Walk instead of driving whenever you can.

- Practice yoga. A regular yoga practice has been linked to a boosted metabolism, weight loss and healthy weight maintenance.

- Stand up every time you answer your phone.

- Smile.

- Laugh more often.

- Reduce the stress in your life. Mental stress leads to physiological changes in your body that promote poor health, and in some cases, weight gain.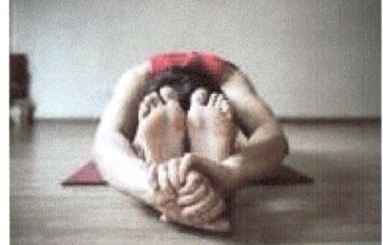

- Try "contrast" showers. This process involves hot water for 2 or 3 minutes, then cold water for 30 to 45 seconds.

- Get at least 6 to 8 hours of sleep each and every night.

- Drink 2 glasses of ice water as soon as you wake up. This is a simple detox process that anyone can benefit from.

Top 10 Reasons Why People Fail to Lose Weight

We just went through how boosting your metabolism can help you lose weight. Now we are going to cover the top reasons why people fail to lose weight. Too many people set out to lose weight and end up failing or giving up. The good news is that being prepared and understanding *why* people fail can help prevent you making the same mistakes. Go through this list, see if any of them sound like something you've done (or not done) and discover how you can overcome these failures so you start losing the weight and keep it off.

#10 Doing a fad diet.

Fad diets don't work. That's the main reason they get coined with the term "fad." They are here today and gone tomorrow. Only healthy eating plans stand the test of time and lose the phrase "fad diet" and become popular and well known.

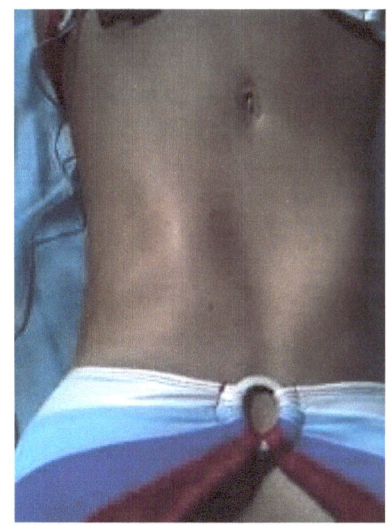

Atkins and South Beach are two that have turned into healthy eating plans. Many doctors and nutritionist are finally coming on board with these two diets.

Following the latest diet craze in the newest edition of some women's magazine is generally not a diet or eating plan you will stick to in the long run. To ensure you have life-long results, you need to make life-long changes in your eating habits.

#9 Eating too few calories.

You know you need to cut calories to lose weight, but restricting your caloric intake too severely will not only have adverse effects on your body, this plan will back fire. A calorie is a unit of fuel. Your body needs fuel to function. When you restrict your daily calorie intake too far below what you need, the body will think it's going into starvation mode and will start taking nutrients from the muscles. You need those muscles. A better approach is to eat the recommended daily calorie allowance for your size and weight loss goals and start adding some muscle building exercises.

Muscles burn fat so adding more muscle will keep your metabolism and the fat burning process going. You may notice a slight increase in weight at first, but keep it up. Before long you'll notice the pounds of fat coming off because the muscles are using that fat as energy/fuel.

#8 Going too long between meals.

Waiting too long to eat can have negative effects in your weight loss process too. The body's metabolism keeps at a good pace as long as it has something to work with. When you skip meals or wait too long the eat, it will slow down your metabolism, thus slowing down the fat burning process as well. It's best to eat several small meals per day, plus have several snacks in between meals. Make sure these are healthy snacks, but eating every few hours will keep your metabolism stoked and ready to go.

#7 Unrealistic weight loss goals.

Setting unrealistic weight loss goals, like expecting to lose ten pounds in one week is another cause of failure. If you don't lose those ten pounds you'll soon give up trying. A better goal is one pound per week. That doesn't sound like much, but over the course of a several weeks or even months it will add up. You didn't put on those extra pounds in a few days, you can't expect to lose them in a few days either. In fact, it may take longer to lose them than it did to gain them. Why? It only takes 2,000 excess calories to put on a pound of weight, but it takes burning 3,500 calories to lose that one pound.

#6 Failing to organize and plan ahead.

Not planning ahead and being organized with your weight loss plans is another cause of failure. If you don't have a plan or a goal to reach, how do you expect to get there? Having a plan means you know when to add an exercise or change up your routine, how many days per week you plan to workout, or even there will be days you need to watch your calories more closely because of a special occasion.

#5 Failing to stock up on the right foods.

If you don't have healthy foods and snacks in your home, you're more likely to grab some junk food when you get hungry. You have to keep good foods on hand so they are available to you at all times. Keep fresh fruits and vegetables well stocked so you can grab those instead of cookies or crackers the next time you want a 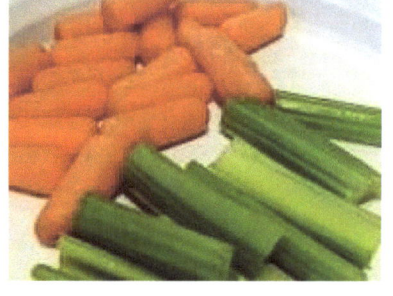 snack. Go ahead and chop some up into bite-sized pieces and keep them in storage containers so you can grab them quickly. This is especially helpful if you've gone too long without eating and need something quick.

#4 Failing to get rid of temptations.

If you keep bad foods around, like chips, cookies, cake or crackers you're more likely to grab those for a quick fix when you get hungry. The old saying, "Out of sight, out of mind," is especially true of food. If you're craving something and it's in your home, chances are you will grab it instead of the fruit or other healthy snacks. Make sure you clean out your pantry before switching to a healthy lifestyle eating plan.

#3 Not exercising.

It doesn't matter how much you cut your calories, you'll get faster results if you exercise. There are many fad diets that claim you can lose weight without exercise, but the truth is the body was designed to move. You don't have to jump into a full-blown fitness guru mode, but you do need to start getting more daily activity into your routine. You can start by walking or doing a light aerobics training a few times each week. It doesn't have to be complicated. Simply start getting out and moving more so you speed up the fat burning process and get your metabolism into a higher gear.

#2 Not having a plan.

This is similar to the one above. If you don't have a plan made out for your weight loss journey you won't have guidelines to stick to. It's much easier to give up if you don't have something written down on your calendar to remind you to get out and exercise or when to increase your exercise. Also, if you plan to introduce new foods into your eating plan, you need 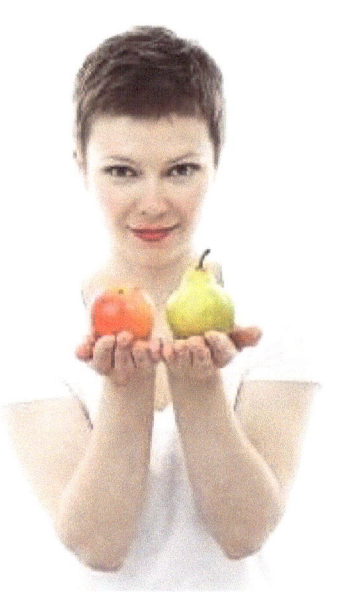 some kind of guide to go by. You may want to add one food per week or one every other week. When you have this written down you don't have to question when or which food it is, you simply look at your plan.

#1 Failing to start.

The number one reason people don't reach weight loss success is that they simply don't start. They keep talking about it, maybe even keep planning it, but until they take action and start working those plans, nothing will happen.

You don't have to start off with starving yourself. You just need to start. You can start by cutting out some junk foods and replacing them with healthier snacks. Start walking 2 or 3 days per week until you can work up to more. The key to success with anything is to start the program. Sticking to it may be hard, but until you start you will not get anywhere.

Don't set yourself up to fail at losing weight. Plan ahead, have healthy, low-fat food at hand, eat regularly and get enough calories so you don't slow down your metabolism, and do the exercise.

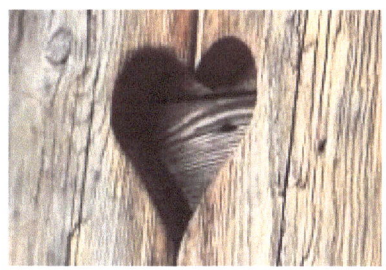

14 Things That Happen After You Lose Weight

When you are overweight, the likelihood that you will contract a chronic disease increases substantially. If you are obese, you have to worry about even more problematic health conditions. The human race is more overweight than ever before. This means you may be looking to drop a few pounds so that you can look and feel better, and improve your health and self-esteem.

If that is the case, good for you.

You are taking your health into your own hands. Reaching and maintaining a healthy body weight is good for so many reasons. However, there may be a few things you didn't consider regarding weight loss. There are some things that happen to your body when you undergo the physiological change of losing weight that you may not have been prepared for, and 14 of the more common side-effects of weight loss (positive and negative) are listed below.

1) You will gain a lot of energy.

You may be losing weight so you will look good in a bikini again. Perhaps all your clothes are getting too tight, and you don't feel like shucking out a couple of thousand dollars for a new, bigger wardrobe. Regardless your reason for losing weight, one thing is certain once you accomplish your goal – you will have a lot more energy.

When you are heavy, all your bodily processes have to work harder. This means that even simple tasks require a lot of energy. It is one of the reasons why overweight and obese individuals often say they 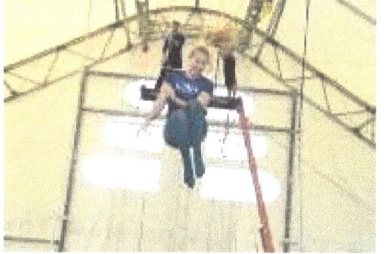 are hungry all of the time. Their body requires more calories to crank out more energy. When you drop your weight, every one of your internal and external processes, from head to toe, gets a break. This makes your organs healthier by not overworking them, and makes more energy available for everyday tasks.

2) Get ready for the backhanded compliments.

"Wow, did you lose weight? You look great!" The first couple of times you hear this, you will probably feel great. Then you realize what the person who told you this might really be saying, "You looked 'not so great' before!"

People often don't think about what they are saying before they open their big mouths. Politely accept the compliments you receive, even if they seem like a double-edged sword.

3) You may lose friends to your new lifestyle.

You lost a bunch of weight, and you look and feel great. Everyone says they are envious of you, and asks how they can get the same results. Don't be surprised if you suggest a trip to the gym, juice shop or health food store and your friends politely decline. Too many people today want results without having to work for them. After you lose weight, you may lose friends to your new, healthier lifestyle.

Some of them may even be abrasive when you turn down unhealthy foods, beverages and habits. Stick to your guns. You worked hard to lose the weight, and gaining it all back just because your friends are lazy or unmotivated is not enough reason to do so.

4) You find out your favorite foods have changed.

Oreos, cheeseburgers, pizza and chocolate-coated anything may not appeal to you after you lose weight. You may not be able to fathom this thought right now.

The fact remains, however, that the physiological process behind significant weight loss can lead you away from unhealthy food addictions to healthier choices.

You will find yourself drawn to fresh fruits and 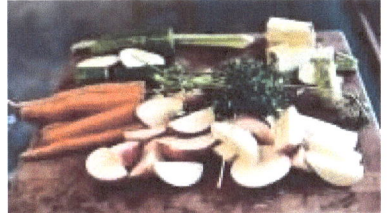 vegetables, healthy juices and smoothies, whole grains, nuts and berries. The thought of a Big Mac, Whopper or Wendy's double may be physically unsettling after you lose weight and reset your taste buds. Fried and fast foods, sugary beverages and energy drinks, baked goods and pastries will begin to take a backseat to healthier food choices.

5) In some people, weight loss can lead to stress.

This doesn't happen to everyone, but it happens enough to mention this side-effect. Doctors will often times tell you to lose weight so that you have less stress in your life. However, if you lose a significant amount of weight in a relatively short period of time, this is a very stressful situation for your body. It could create hormonal changes that lead to an overproduction of cortisol, nicknamed the stress hormone. If you find your weight loss leading to mental stress and anxiety, consult your physician.

6) Your breasts may shrink.

Men will probably love this, and women may not. Breasts, in both men and women, growth in size due to fat storage. Men with man boobs will absolutely love the fact that weight loss can lead to a reduction in the size of their breasts. Women may or may not enjoy the fact that their breasts become smaller, depending on personal preference and any relevant health conditions. Don't forget that you can't "spot reduce" fat in one area, and not lose fat in another.

7) You are going to need to spend some money.

Let's face it, if you lose any significant amount of weight, your current clothes are not going to fit properly. This means an entire new wardrobe to show off your slim, sexy, confident body. You may also have to purchase healthy lifestyle influences like juicers, mixers and exercise equipment. So be prepared to slide the plastic after you lose the desired amount of weight and hit your target number.

8) You become an exercise freak!

Oh, you don't think so right now. When you see those pounds starting to drop off, your attitude may change.

Even though you used to dread working out, after you lose some weight start to see the results, you might become one of those people who gets addicted to healthy exercise and wants to work out as frequently as possible.

9) You can finally keep up with your kids/grandchildren.

A lot of people attempt to lose weight so they can spend more time with the people they love. In many cases, however, your kids just have way more energy than you do. If your children are grown, the disparity between your energy level and that of your grandchildren is probably even more pronounced.

One wonderful side-effect of losing weight and becoming healthy is that your body is stronger, more capable and flexible, and you have more energy.

This means you can create wonderful memories with your children and grandchildren, without feeling pooped and out of breath after just a few minutes of play.

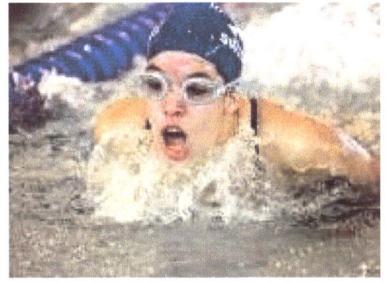

10) Your children become healthier.

Kids look up to their parents. You may be losing weight for your own personal reasons. Fortunately, because children are sponges and absorb everything they see and hear, after you start 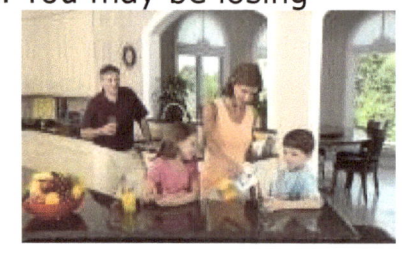 losing weight, your kids may want to jump on the bandwagon. This is one of the most rewarding and positive side-effects of healthy weight loss.

11) You feel colder than normal.

After you lose weight, you don't have as much fat to insulate your body from external temperatures. This means you will be more sensitive to colder temperatures than you were when you were overweight. You may find yourself needing a jacket or coat when previously you didn't. On the positive side, your air conditioning costs may go down because you don't have to keep your home as cold as you used to.

12) People turn to you as a weight loss "guru".

This could be good ... or bad. You are probably going to want to spread the word about your weight loss journey. No doubt your friends, family members and coworkers will notice how slim, trim, healthy and happy you look and feel.

If they are overweight, it is only natural that they will ask you how you gained the results you're looking for.

This is great, because you are acting as a positive role model. The problem is when you tell someone exactly what you did, they do the same, and see very little to no results. Everyone is different, from metabolism to motivation to action and consistency of efforts. Be proud the people are looking at you as a positive influence, while simultaneously reminding those that ask for weight loss advice that they may get different results than you did.

13) You will not be able to stop looking at yourself in a mirror.

This may seem a little egotistical, but honestly, go ahead and take a long look. You worked very hard to lose the weight, and there is nothing wrong with being proud about what you have accomplished. Just don't be 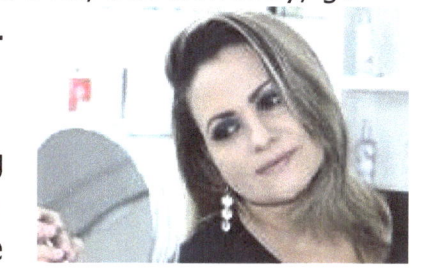 that person that gets caught in public checking themselves out in every available mirror and reflective shop window.

14) You live a longer and healthier life.

It's funny. When people stress about losing weight, focusing on a particular number of pounds to lose, or a target body weight, weight loss seems to be very difficult. They try every possible diet and exercise plan and struggle to lose weight. On the other hand, if you just eat right, exercise, drink plenty of water and get lots of rest, weight loss and a healthy body weight maintenance comes naturally.

Why is that?

Is because your body weight is simply a factor resulting from a physiological formula. When you give your body the proper nutrients, minerals and vitamins it needs, all of your intricate and amazing external and internal processes work perfectly. Add exercise to burn fat and calories, while building healthy muscle, and you become even healthier and more resistant to illness, disease and infection.

Conclusion?

The lesson here is to focus on living a healthy lifestyle, and your weight loss will take care of itself. Without the pressure of having to eat a certain way or o lose a set amount of weight in a specified time, the pressure is off and you can lose weight at your own schedule.

With "diets", there is an ending point because most of them are so restrictive that you can't stay on them forever. By choosing a healthy lifestyle there is no ending point; it is something you will do forever. The only change that will happen is once you reach your weight goal, you'll add in a few more calories per day to stay at that weight. If you are still losing, add in more calories. If you start gaining, cut back a little on calories or increase your exercising to burn more calories.

Losing weight is simply a numbers game – burn more calories than you take in. Eighty percent of losing weight is through nutrition; 20% is from exercising. However as shown, exercising – especially strength training – builds muscle mass which increases your metabolism to keep the extra muscle functioning throughout the day (and even at night while you sleep).

Other Senior Health and Fitness Books by This Author

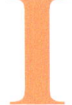f you would like to read more about Senior Health and Fitness, here is a list of the <u>titles, CreateSpace links and descriptions:</u>

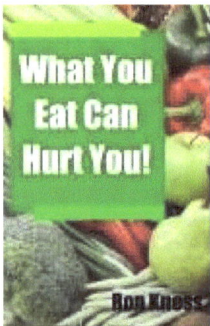

[What You Eat Can Hurt You](#)

https://www.createspace.com/4963196

Do you know that certain foods increase your risk for inflammation, disease and illness? It's true! And certain foods can help cure and heal you if you do get sick. Knowing which foods to eat and which ones to avoid empowers you to manage your own health.

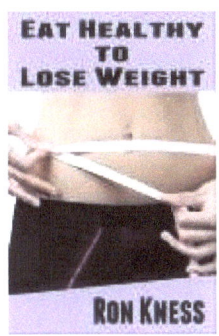 [Eat Healthy to Lose Weight](#)

https://www.createspace.com/4962939

As you read through our book, we show you which foods you should and should not be eating to reach your weight loss goal, along with discussing how to maintain your weight loss and stay within a few pounds of your goal weight. Banish the weight you keep gaining back each time by learning how to live a healthy lifestyle.

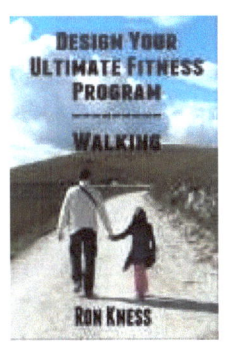 [Design Your Ultimate Fitness Program - Walking](#)

https://www.createspace.com/5252272

In my book Design Your Ultimate Fitness Program – Walking, we discuss the considerations that need to be made when designing a custom walking program, along with:
• Equipment needed

• Wearable technology you can use to track your walking
• And how to make walking more challenging

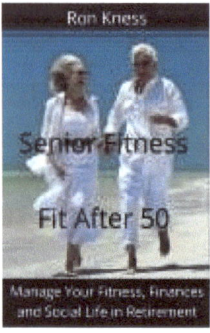

Senior Fitness – Fit After 50: Learn How to Manage Your Fitness, Finances and Social Life in Retirement

https://www.createspace.com/5474751

Inside you will discover answers to your most pressing questions:
• What do I need to know about downsizing my home?
• What are the best tips for staying healthy as you approach your 50's?
• When should I start planning for retirement?
• I am worried about being lonely once I retire, do others feel the same?
• Is it worthwhile to carry two homes during retirement?
And more…

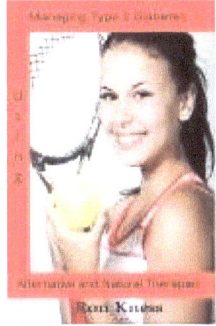

Managing Type 2 Diabetes Using Alternative And Natural Therapies

https://www.createspace.com/5401244

While Type 2 diabetes can be managed medically, there are many alternative natural and holistic methods of therapy and treatment that can further enhance quality of life and minimize the effects of this disease. In this book, I discuss 12 different types, including yoga, reflexology and acupuncture to name just three.

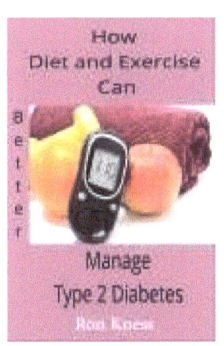

How Diet and Exercise Can Better Manage Type 2 Diabetes

https://www.createspace.com/5404845

Of the different types of diabetes, only Type 2 can be reversed. In my book How Diet and Exercise Can Better Manage Type 2 Diabetes, we reveal the three things you can do to best manage your disease, including:
• Diet

- Exercise
- Weight management

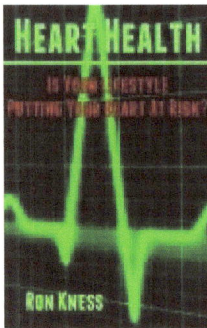

Heart Health: Is Your Lifestyle Putting Your Heart at Risk?

https://www.createspace.com/5464020

In my ebook Is Your Lifestyle Putting Your Heart At Risk? we discuss the six greatest risks to your heart and the lifestyle changes you can make to mitigate them.

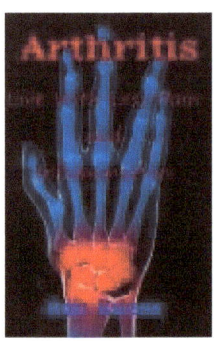

Arthritis – Live Wth Less Pain and Inflammation: Tips and Techniques You Can Use to Lessen the Pain and Inflammation

https://www.createspace.com/5457441

Discover Simple Tips & Information That Will Help Reduce The Painful Symptoms Of Arthritis!

You learn things like:

• Simple and effective information that will help you manage the pain and inflammation that comes along with arthritis, so that you can live an active, full life without debilitating pain.

• The different types of arthritis, their symptoms and how to alleviate their painful side effects.

• The pros and cons of over-the-counter arthritis medications, plus simple tips that will help you know how to choose the right supplements.

• Free, yet effective ways to get relief from arthritis pain and inflammation, so you don't have to suffer anymore.

the effects arthritis can have significant impact on your physical and mental well-being, but this books shows you how to overcome its painful symptoms and live life relatively pain free.

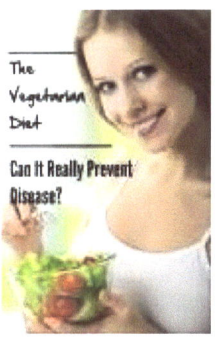

The Vegetarian Diet – Can It Really Prevent Disease?

https://www.createspace.com/5519874

Is a vegetarian diet right for you? Multiple studies have shown over and over that a vegetarian diet goes along way in preventing certain chronic diseases, such as:

• Heart Disease
• Cancer
• Diverticulitis
• Type 2 Diabetes

- Hypertension
- Obesity
- Kidney Failure

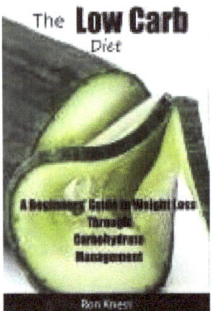

The Low Carb Diet: A Beginner's Guide to Weight Loss Through Carbohydrate Management

https://www.createspace.com/5416348

In my book "The Low-Carb Diet – A Beginners' Guide to Weight Loss Through Carbohydrate Management", I reveal a successful method of losing weight based in part on the amount and type of carbohydrates you consume.

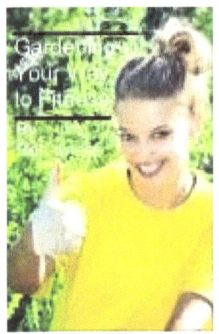

Gardening Your Way to Fitness: The Fun Way to Get Fit and Provide Beauty and Healthful Bounty for Your Family

https://www.createspace.com/5459564

The gym is a great place to stay fit during the colder seasons, but once the temperature turns warmer you want to spend more time outside. Plus, you'll have the benefit of fresh wholesome produce to enjoy by growing vegetables in your backyard garden.

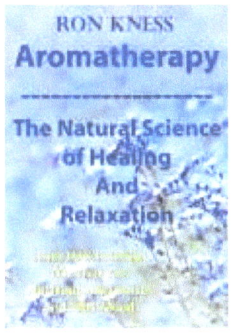

Aromatherapy - The Science of Healing and Relaxation: Learn How Essential Oils Elicit The Relaxation Response And Alter Mood

https://www.createspace.com/5714434

In my book Aromatherapy – The Science of Healing and Relaxation, we reveal the natural holistics methods you can use to heal the body from certain medical issues and to relive stress through relaxation. In particular we talk about:
• Aromatherapy - what it is and how it works
• Essential Oils – how the effects of certain aromas differs from others
• Recipes – how to make your own essential oil combinations

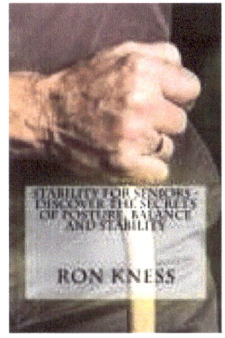

Stability for Seniors: Discover the Secrets of Posture, Balance and Stability

https://www.createspace.com/6096479

Many people sacrifice their health in pursuit of their career. They are so busy making a living that they neglect to make a life. The excuse that they do not have time to exercise is tossed about so frequently that they end up letting their health and fitness slide.

If you are not regularly active, you will have muscular atrophy over time. Your flexibility will decrease. Your core strength will diminish. As time progresses, you will be less limber and more rigid.

This is exactly how people age poorly. It's a process that has snowballed over time.

Only with regular exercise and a healthy diet can you have a body that is fit and has the ability to almost reverse aging.

If you have neglected your health for years and life seems to be a chore now because you can't get around without assistance, do not feel dejected.

You can remedy the situation. You can restore the strength, balance and stamina that you have lost. It is never too late to become what you might have been.

This guide will show you exactly what you need to do to restore your balance, strengthen your core and give you the ability to live life to its fullest. Read how …

About the Author

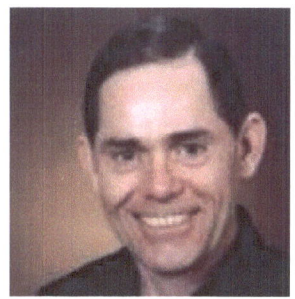

I grew up in Central Minnesota, where my parents owned and operated a fishing resort. Once out of high school I tried a couple of semesters of college, only to quit halfway through the Spring term; I decided at that time that college wasn't for me.

Then I decided to follow my father's previous occupation as an auto mechanic. I graduated from a two-year of vocational training course and worked as a mechanic. While in vocational training, I decided to join the National Guard where I eventually ended up working full-time for 32 years.

So how does all of this relate to writing? In one of my leadership schools, the instructor, who was an English teacher at a juvenile detention center, presented writing to me in a whole new way - a way that started to develop my interest in working with words.

Fast forward about 40 years and I now have over 50 books listed on Amazon for Kindle and CreateSpace.

Besides my own writing, I also ghostwrite ebooks, reports, articles, blogs and do Kindle conversions for my clients on a variety of topics.

Today my wife and I live in Gold Canyon, AZ, where you'll find me happily sitting in my office typing away on my laptop as I work on my next book or ghostwriting project . . . that is if we are not traveling on a cruise ship - our new-found mode of travel.

www.ingramcontent.com/pod-product-compliance
Lightning Source LLC
Chambersburg PA
CBHW050826290526
45792CB00001B/277